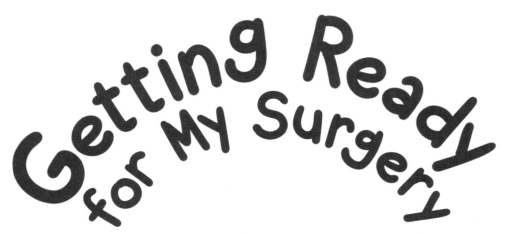

Getting Ready for My Surgery

Preparing Kids for Anesthesia

This book belongs to:

D1613813

Written by Dr. Fei Zheng-Ward   Illustrated by Moch. Fajar Shobaru

Copyright © 2024 Fei Zheng-Ward

Identifiers: ISBN 979-8-89318-006-0 (eBook)
ISBN 979-8-89318-007-7 (paperback)

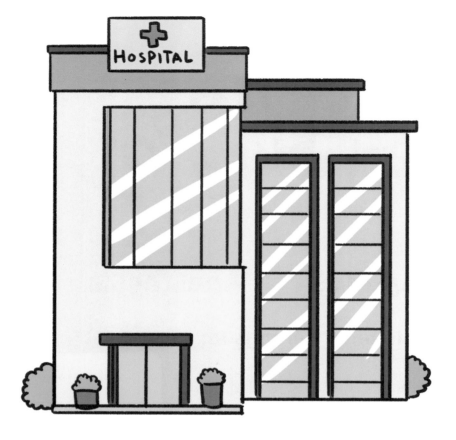

On the day of your surgery, you will arrive at the hospital.

You can bring your favorite toy or blanket.

You may feel a little scared; that's OK.

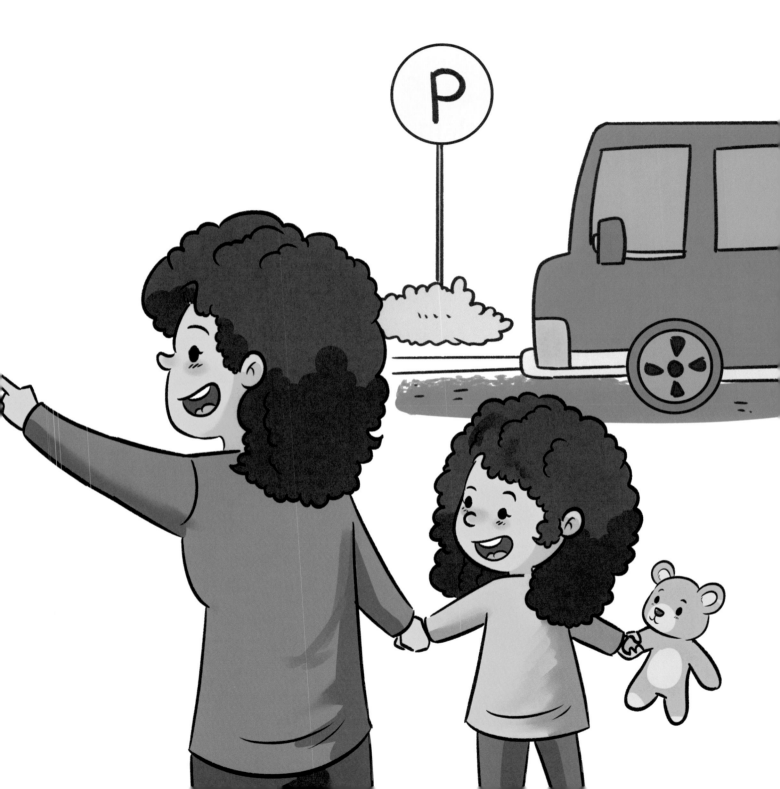

You will check in at the hospital and give them your name and birth date.

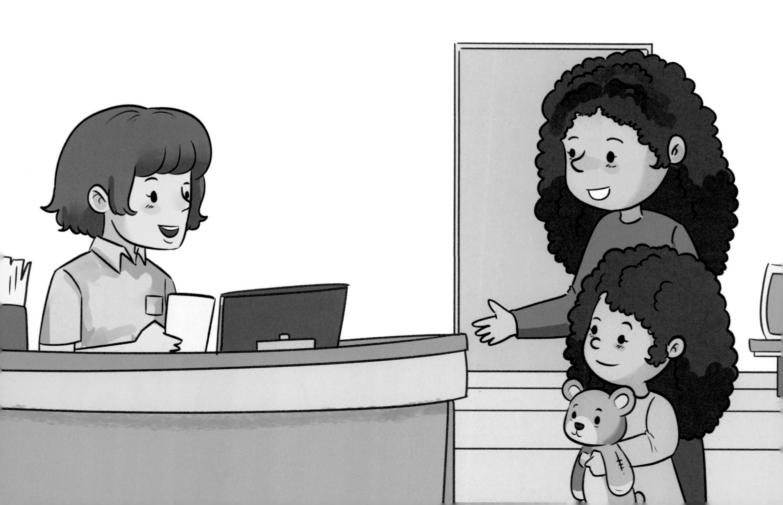

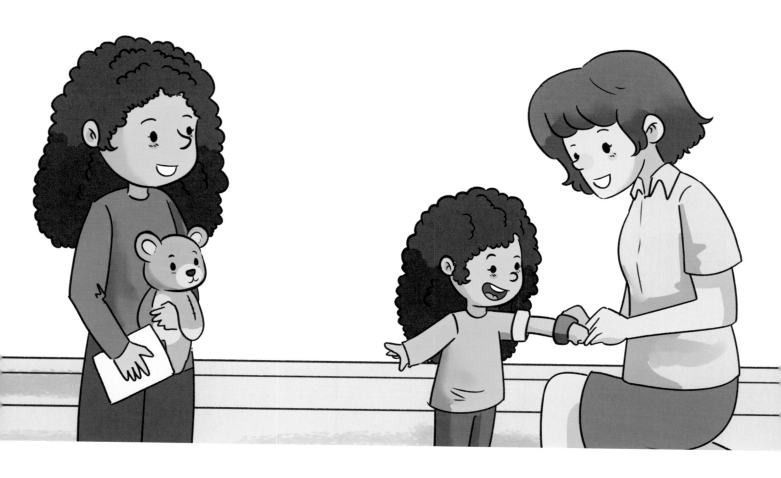

Then, you will receive a special wristband.
Now everyone will know your name.

What color wristband will you get?

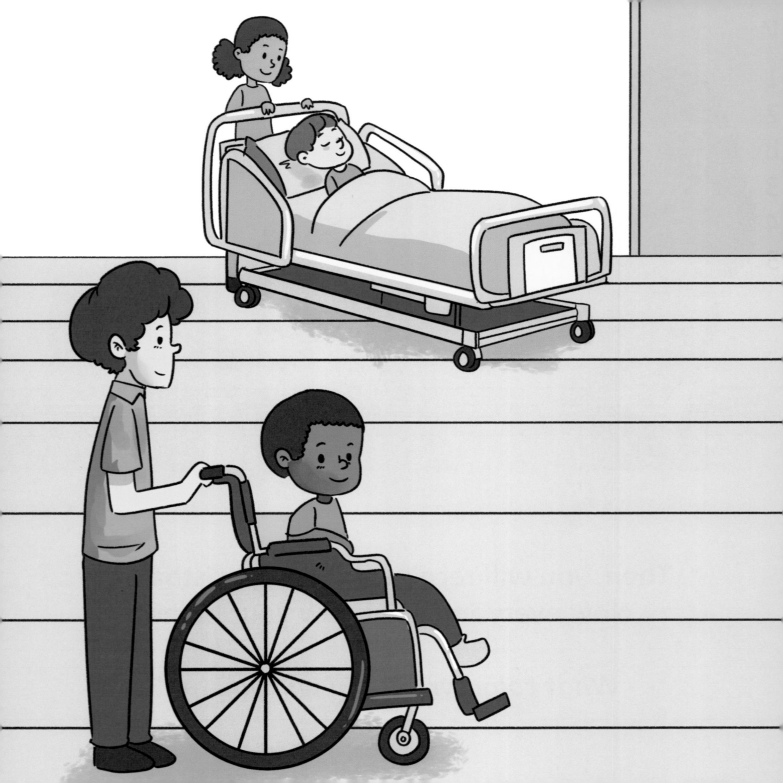

While at the hospital, can you spot the following items?

1. White coat
2. Stethoscope (used to listen to your heart, lungs, and belly)
3. Gloves
4. Bed on wheels
5. Wheelchair

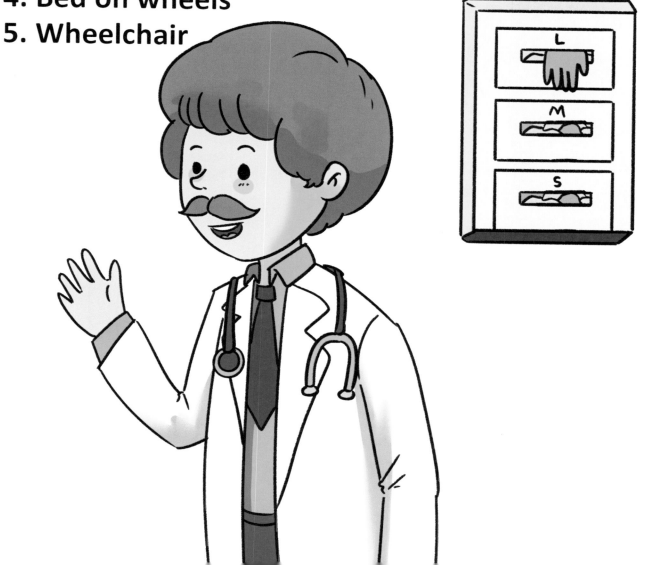

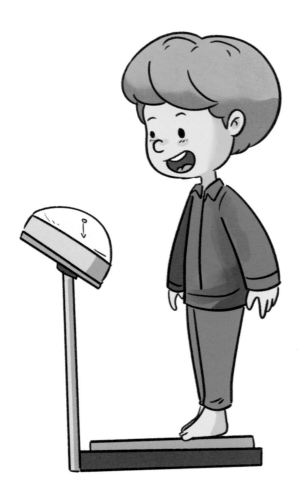

They will check your weight and height before getting you ready.

Do you know how much you weigh?

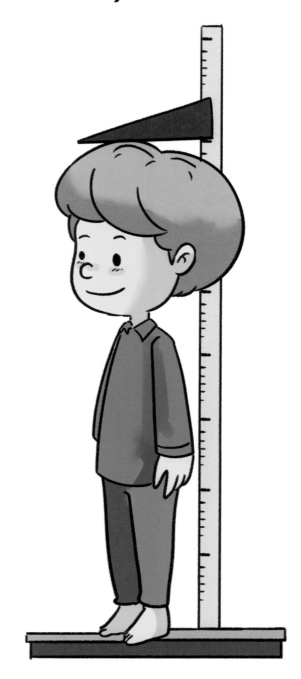

Do you know how tall you are?

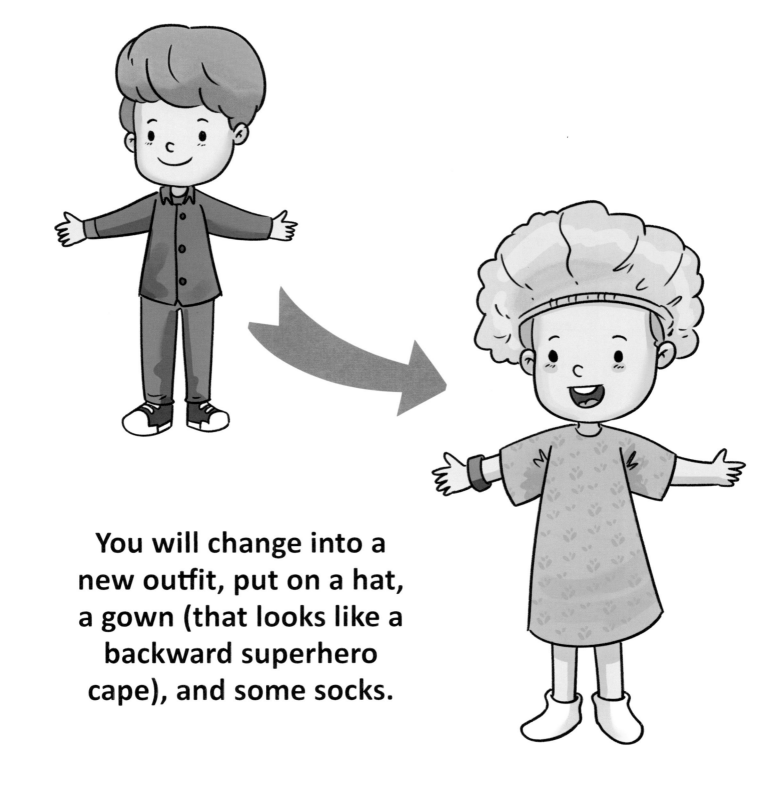

You will change into a
new outfit, put on a hat,
a gown (that looks like a
backward superhero
cape), and some socks.

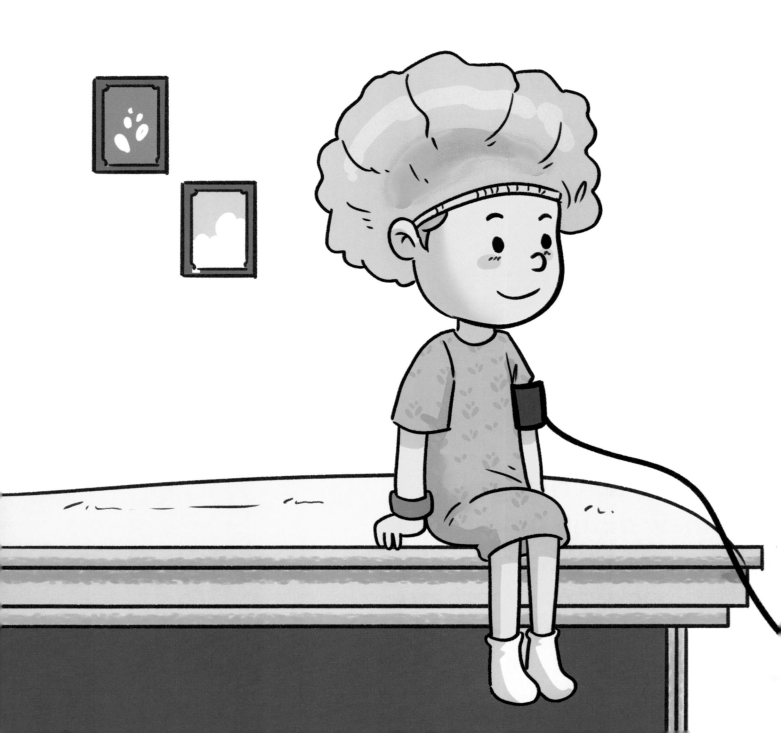

The nurse will put a blood pressure cuff around your arm or leg. The cuff will give you a **BIG** squeeze.

Don't forget to stay still while they're examining you.

Are you ready?

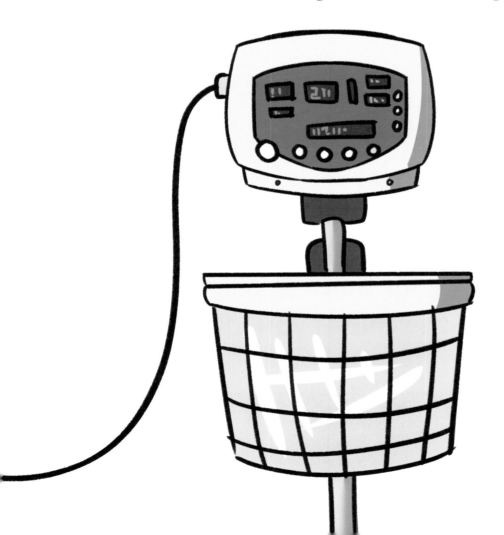

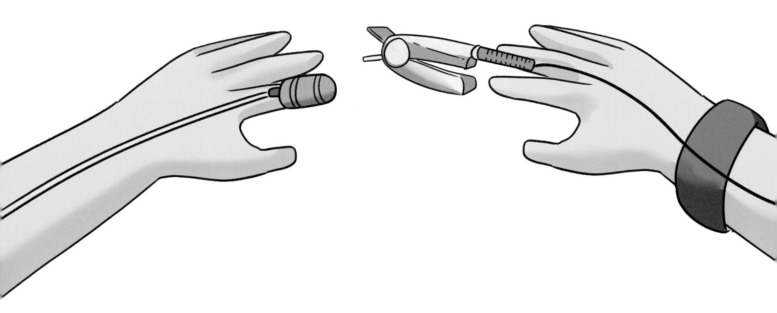

Your nurse will put a bandage-like tape or a clip on your finger or toe to see how much oxygen is in your body.

Oxygen keeps your body working so you can do the things you love.

Which finger or toe do you want to use?

Your friendly anesthesia and surgery doctors will come to talk to you.

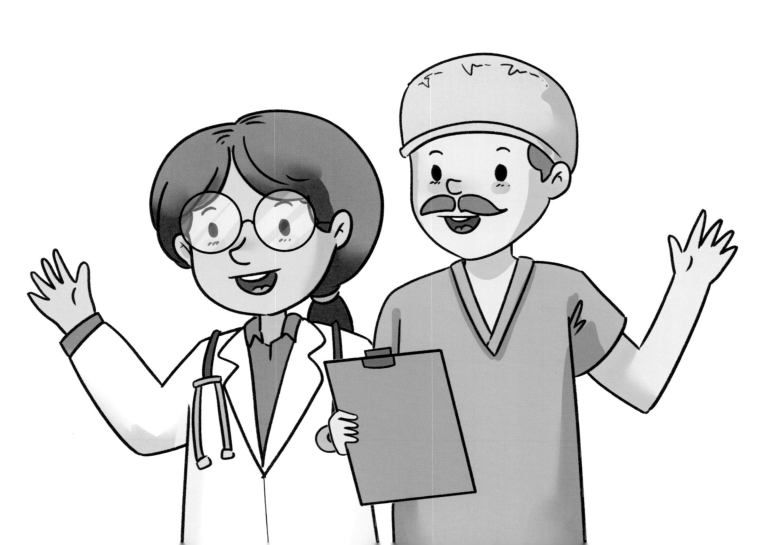

They may listen to your heart, lungs, and belly to make sure you stay healthy.

If you have any questions for your doctors and nurses, please write them down below.

_____

_____

_____

_____

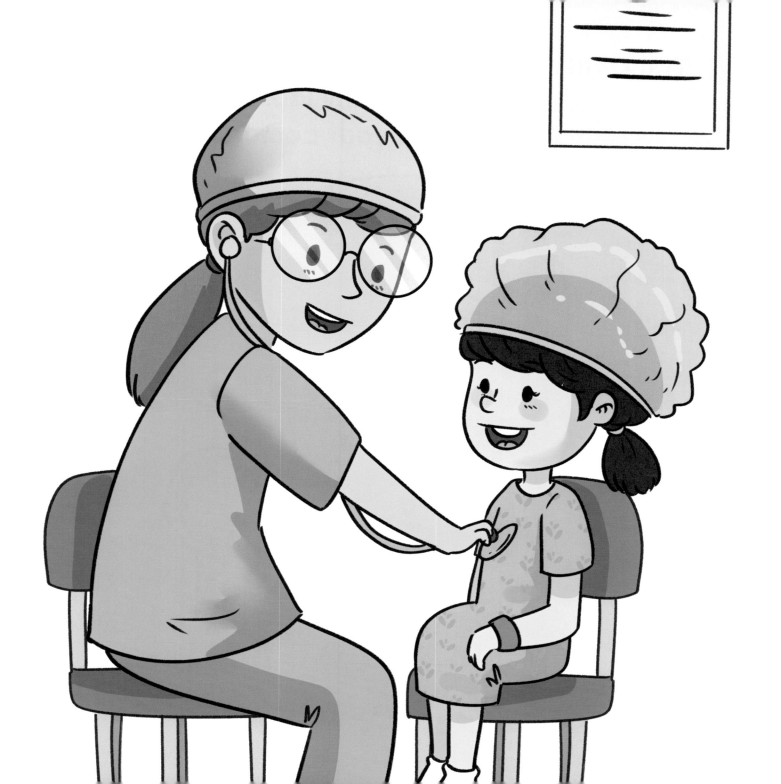

They will even check your teeth and have you say, "Aaah." If you have any loose teeth, don't forget to tell your doctors.

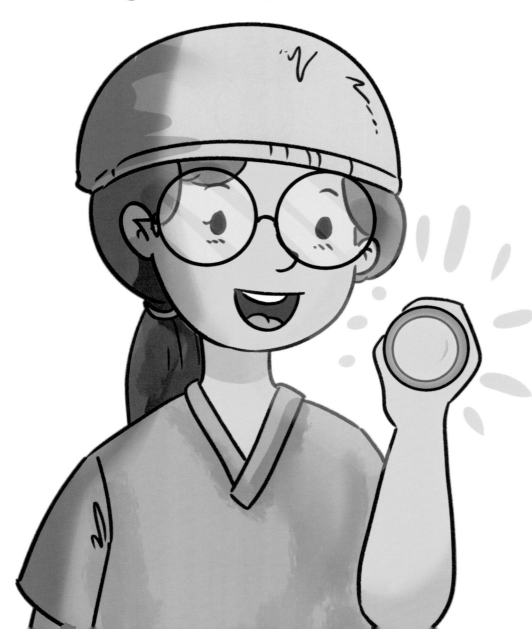

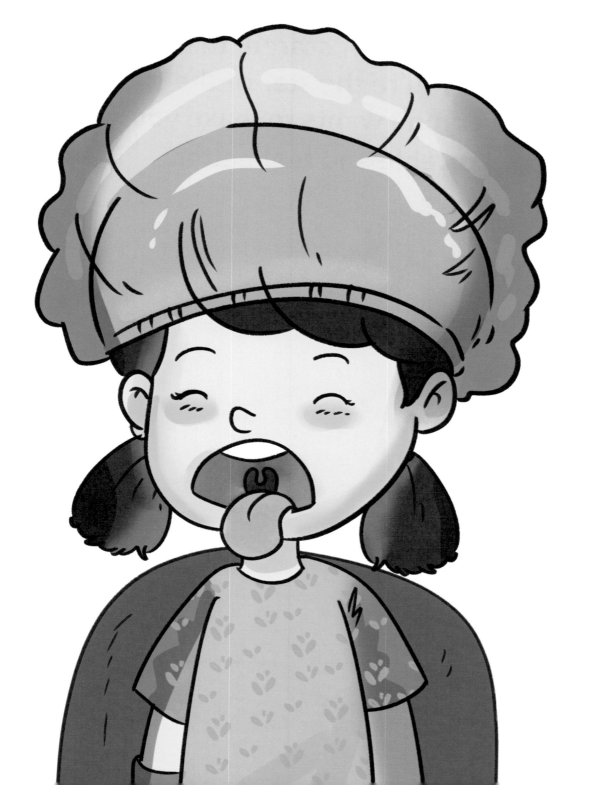

If you get nervous or scared, that's OK. Remember, you're the star of the show, and everyone wants to make you comfortable and feel better.

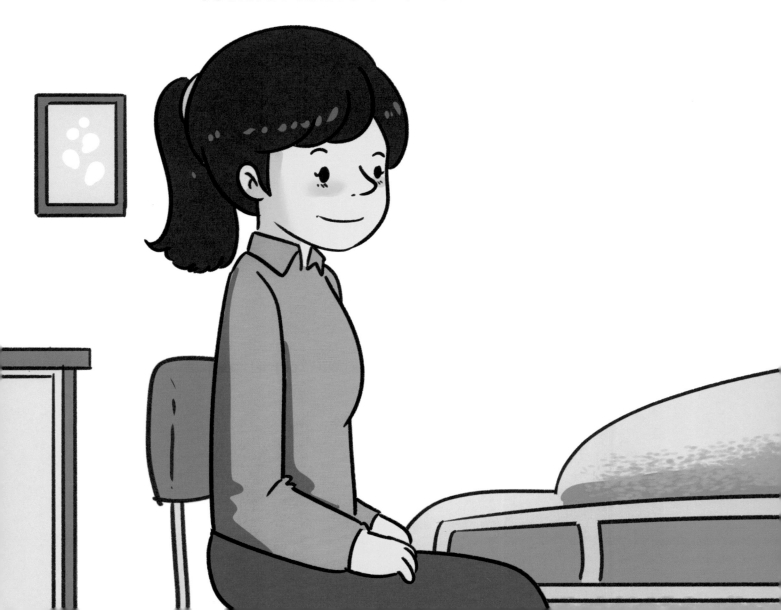

You may get a special, sweet medicine
to help you feel more calm.

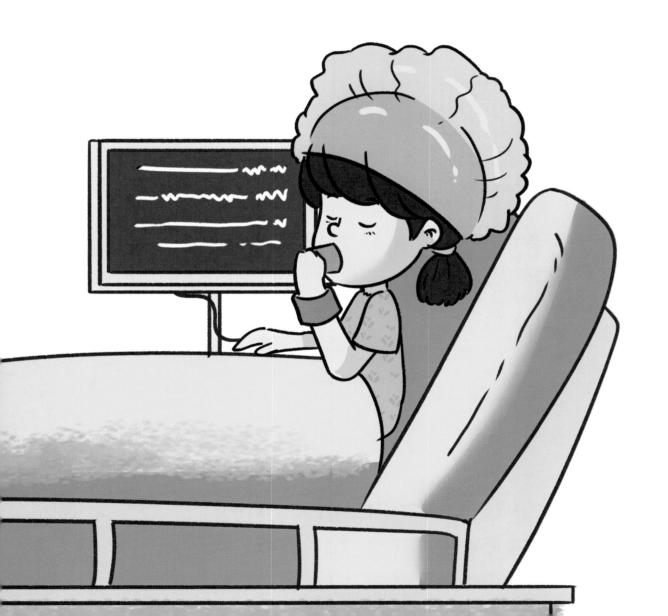

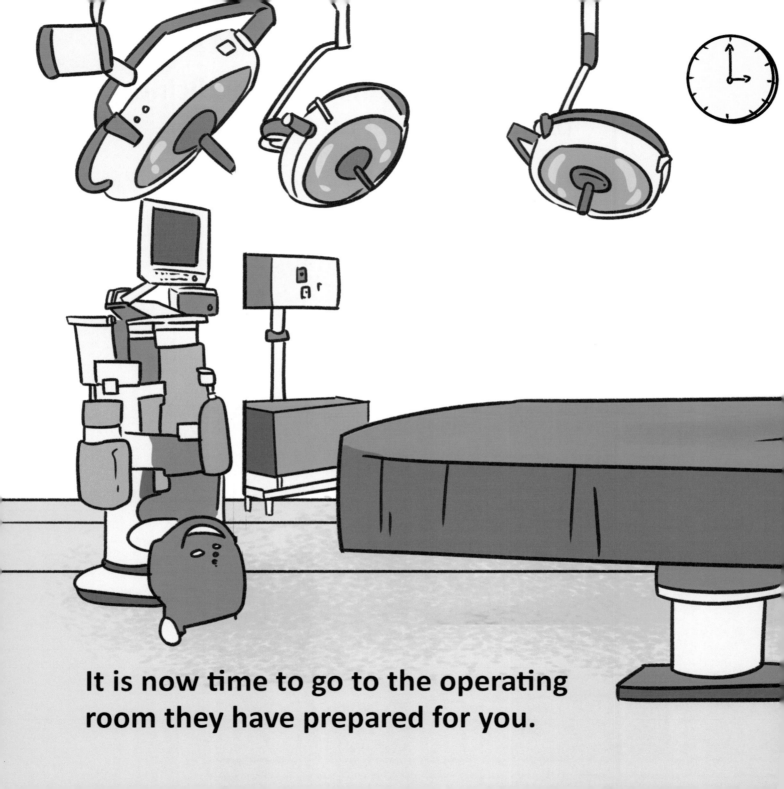

It is now time to go to the operating
room they have prepared for you.

Can you spot the following items in the room?

1. Bright lights hanging from the ceiling
2. People wearing masks
3. A warm bed in the room just for you
4. Computer
5. Clock

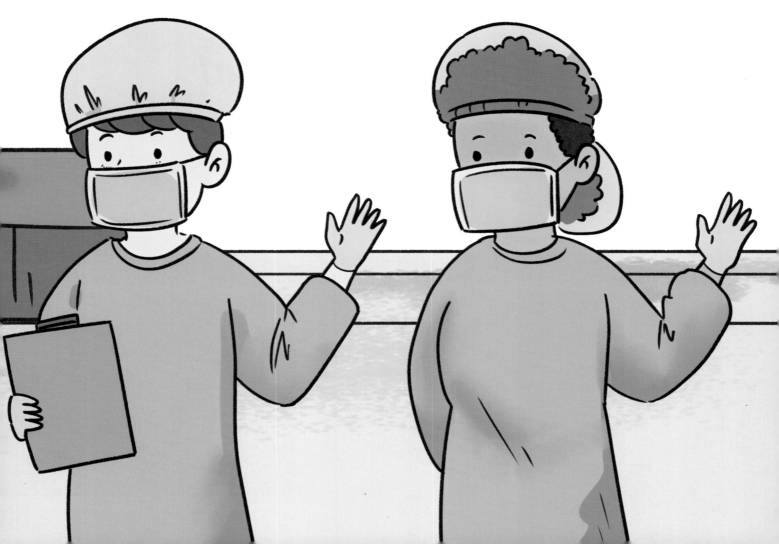

After you get on the bed in the center of the room, they will check your heart, lungs, breathing, and blood pressure once again.

You are so brave!

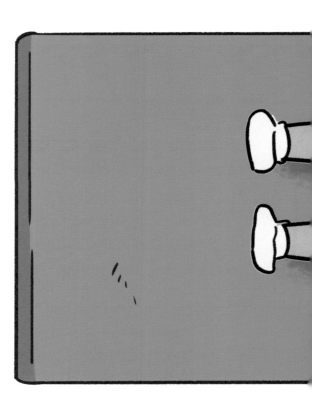

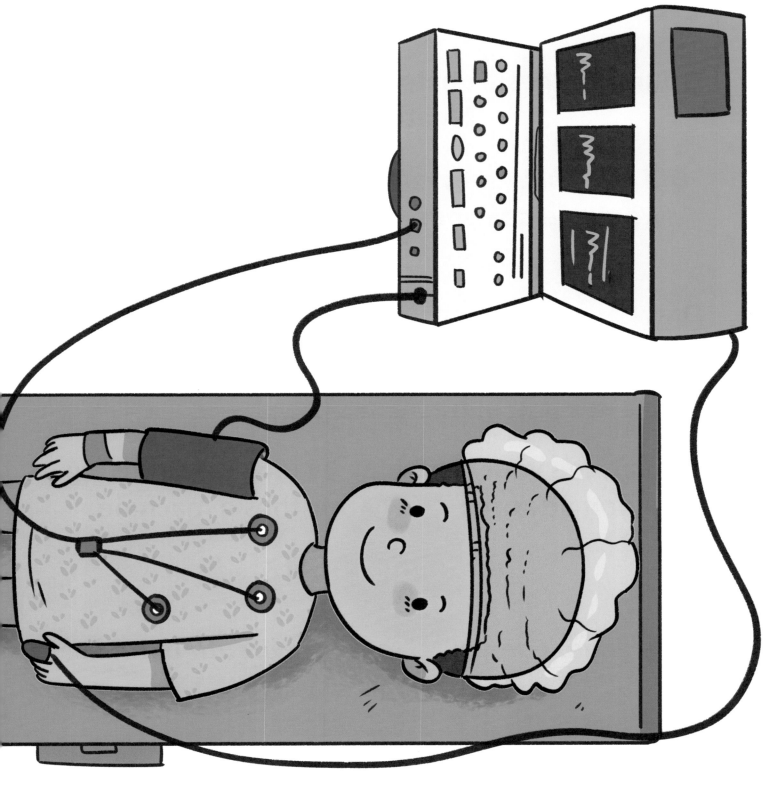

Your anesthesia doctor will give you a mask to breathe into.

Did you know they can make your mask smell sweet and delicious like bubble gum or your favorite fruit?

Draw or write down what scent you would like:

_____

You can see your breathing by looking at the big balloon attached to the anesthesia machine.

Pretty cool, right?

*Challenge: Can you take a **BIG** breath to make the balloon smaller?*

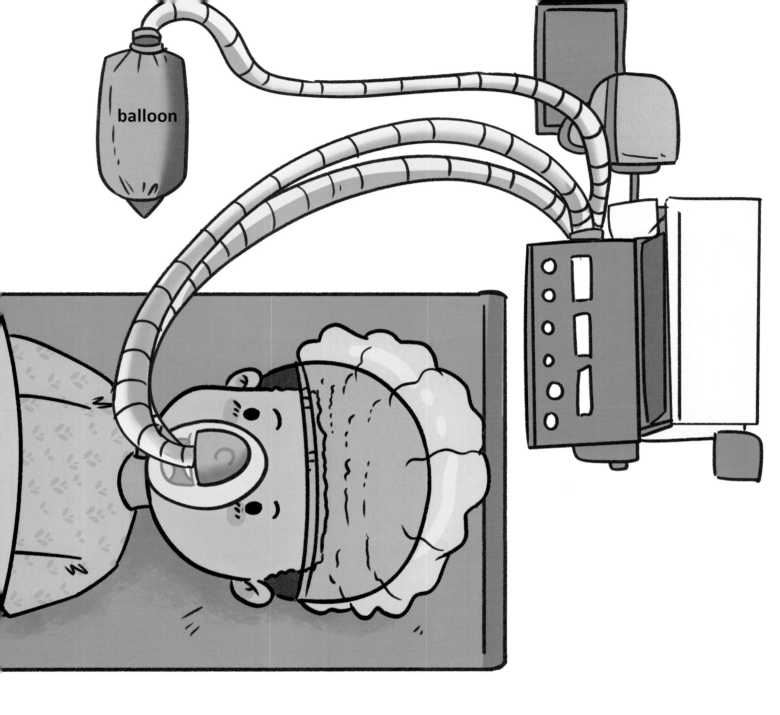

Your medical team will give you "laughing gas" to breathe.

Do you know why it is called "laughing gas?"

Because it makes you *laugh!*

So, laugh and don't hold back.

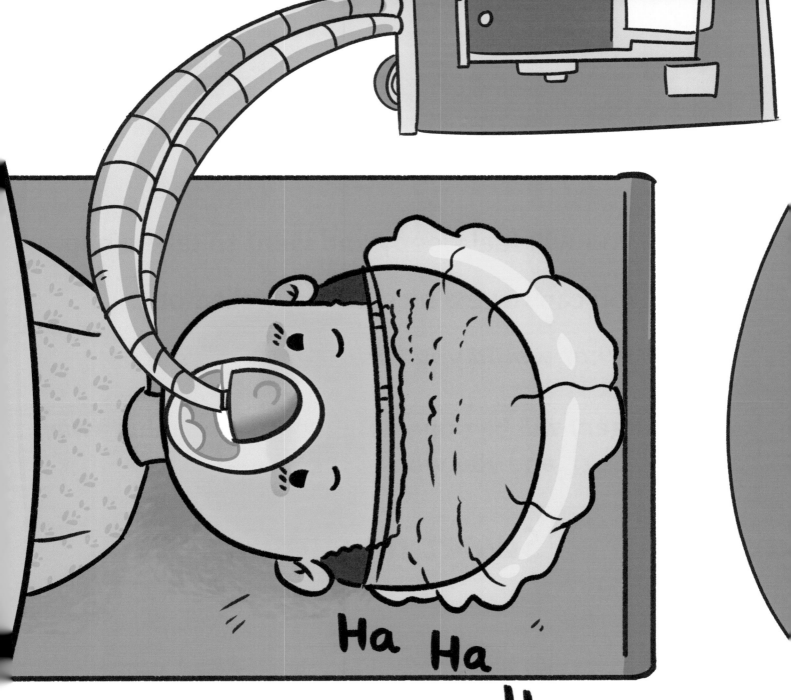

Soon, you will feel sleepy and want to take a nap.

You can have a nice dream picked out.

What would you like to dream about?

Your surgery will be done while you're dreaming away, and you won't feel a thing!

Sweet dreams...

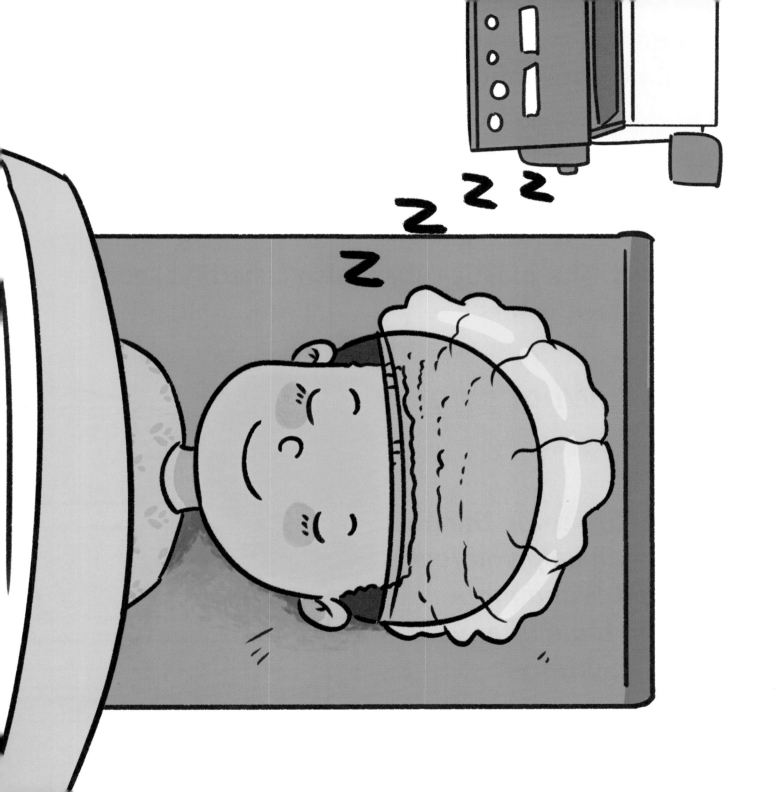

When you wake up from your nap, your surgery will be done, and you may be uncomfortable.

But don't worry, you will get special medicine to make you feel better. It will be given to you through the small plastic tube in your arm or leg. The tube was placed when you were sleeping.

Fun fact: The plastic tubes (also called IVs) come in different colors like yellow, blue, pink, green, gray, and orange.

What color will you get?

What are some things that will help you feel better and more comfortable after your surgery?

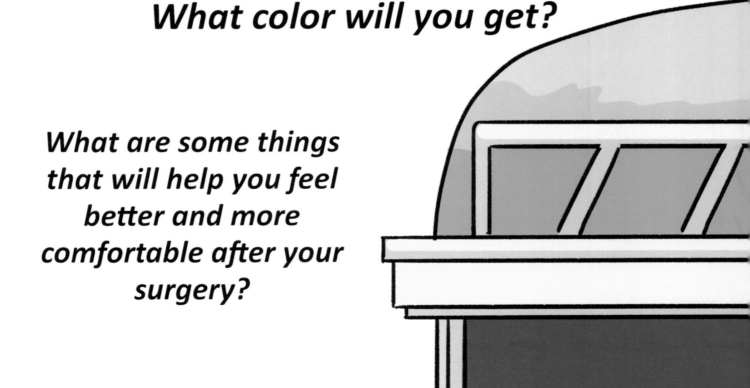

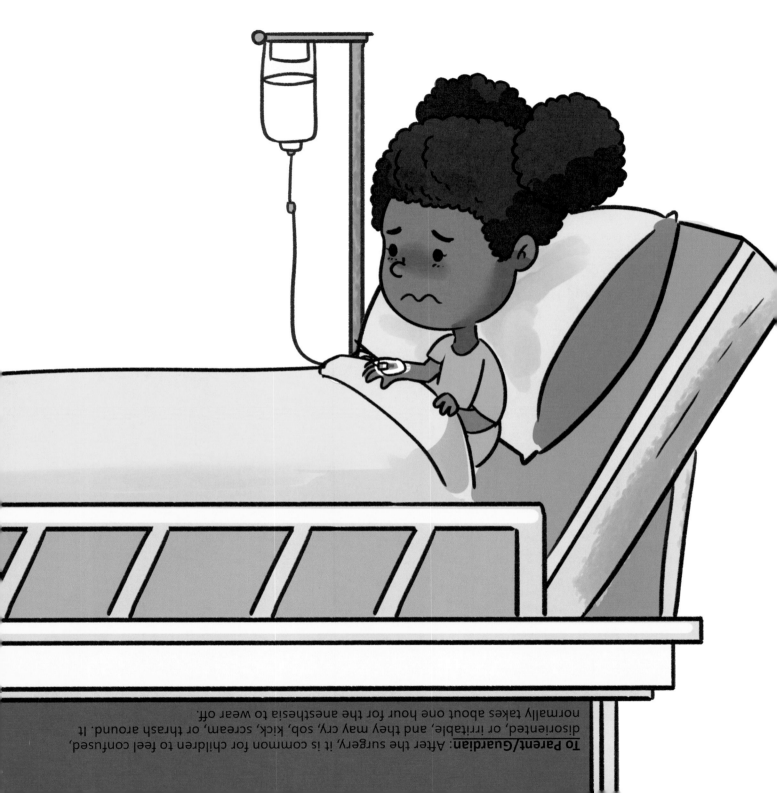

Everyone will see how brave you have been.

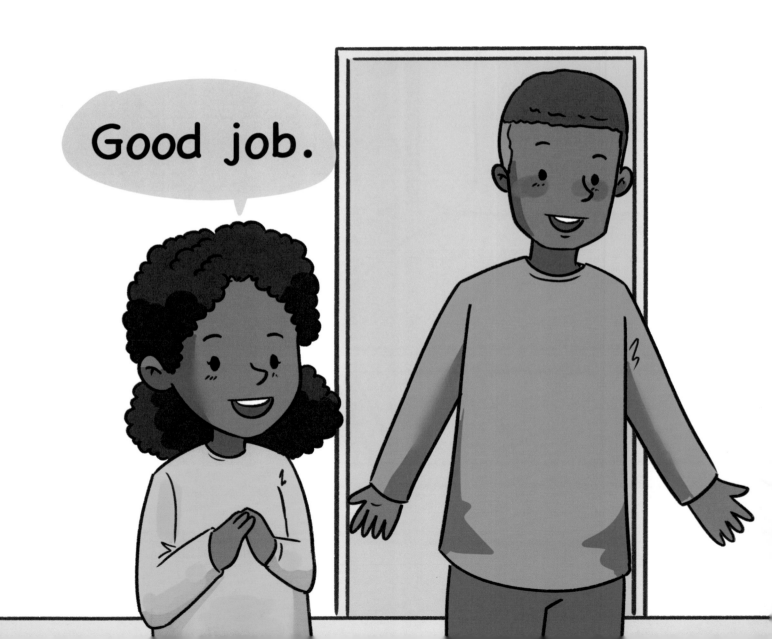

When you feel well enough, you can get some juice or a snack.

What do you want to eat after your surgery?

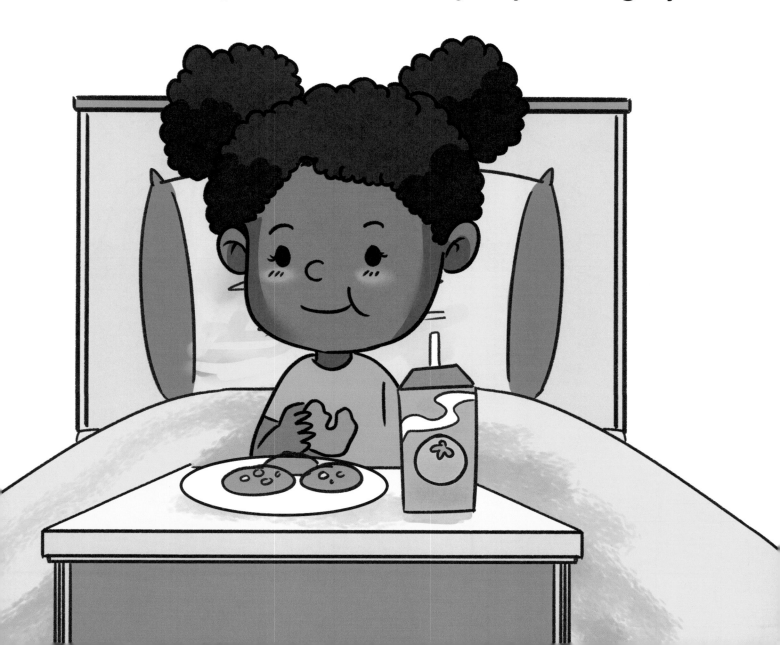

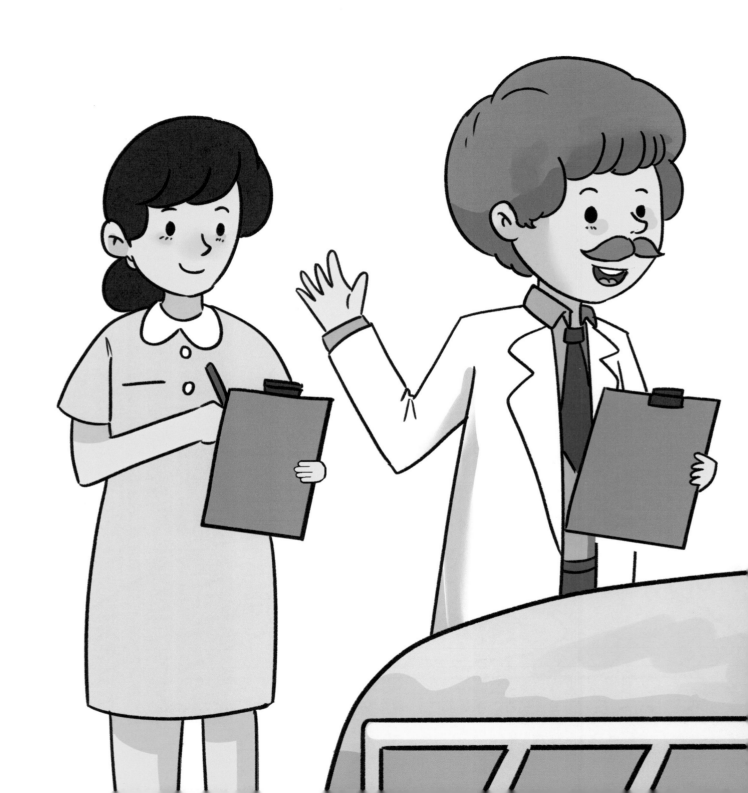

Sometimes, you may have to stay in the hospital after your surgery.

Your parent or guardian can stay with you.

Your doctors and nurses will keep you safe and comfortable.

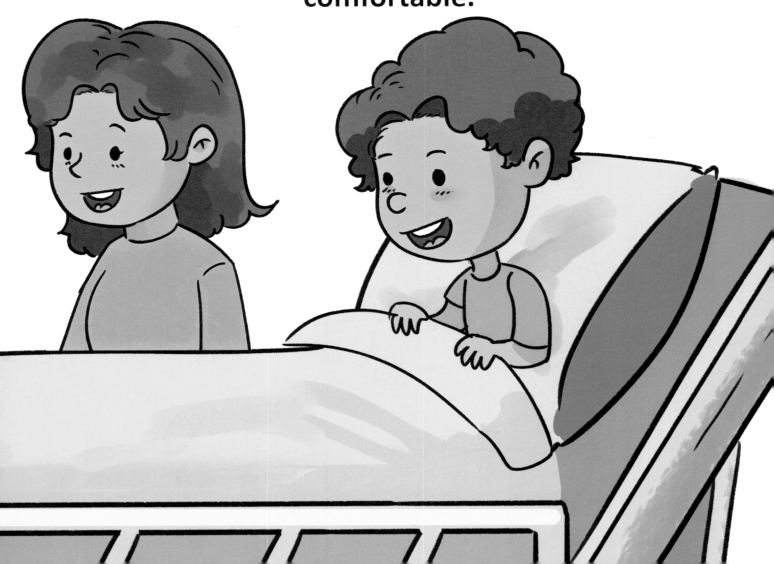

Before you know it, it will be time to go home.
Your adventure at the hospital is almost over.

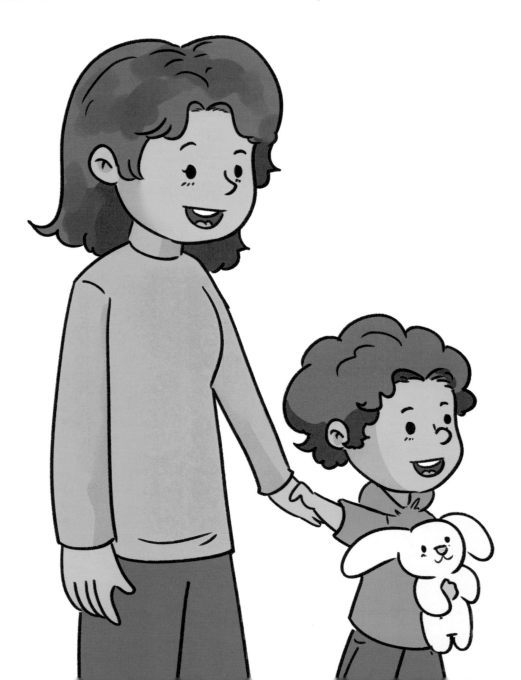

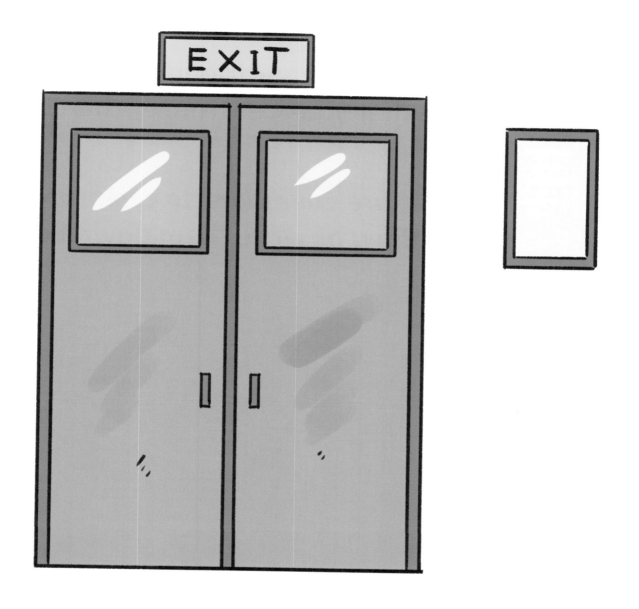

I hope you had some fun exploring it while you were there for your surgery.

Now you can tell your friends how brave you were and that you are stronger than before.

What are your plans to celebrate?
Please draw or write them down below.

Speedy recovery!

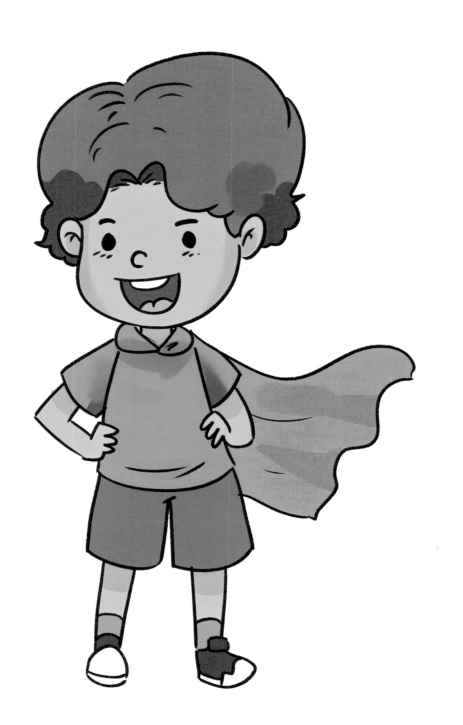

Notes for Parent/Guardian

Here is a list of foods and liquids and their corresponding times that need to pass between the time your child finishes eating or drinking them and the start of their surgery (from the American Society of Anesthesiologists):

Full meal or fatty foods: 8 hours
Infant formula or animal/plant milk: 6 hours
Breast milk: 4 hours
Clear liquids: 2 hours

Clear liquids are see-through liquids and some examples are apple juice (*not* apple cider), water, sugar water, and Pedialyte (*not* PediaSure). Orange juice is *not* a clear liquid.

Please note that every child is different, and it is important to discuss and confirm the above recommendations with your child's doctor prior to the day of surgery.
* If your child takes medicines regularly, please ask their doctor for instructions regarding the medicines for before and after the surgery.
* Placement of intravenous (IV) catheter in this young age group is typically done _after_ your child is asleep in the operating or procedure room.
* Marking of the surgical site by the surgeon may or may not apply to your child depending on the type of surgery or procedure and its laterality (left, right, or both sides).
* Depending on the type of surgery, your child may or may not have a visible scar.

Disclaimer

Please note that the illustrations are not drawn to scale.

This book is written for informational, educational, and personal growth purposes and should not be used as a substitute for medical advice.

Please consult your child's doctor if they need medical attention and to ensure the information in this book pertains to your child's medical condition and needs. I cannot guarantee what your child experiences is exactly what is being discussed in this book.

The author and the publisher are not responsible, either directly or indirectly, for any damages, monetary loss, or reparation due to information in this book. By reading this book, the readers agree not to hold the author and the publisher responsible for any losses as a result of any errors, inaccuracies, or omissions in this book.

Please keep in mind that your child's experience depends on the location, the facility, their medical condition, and the healthcare team. Please use this book in conjunction with your child's doctor's advice. Thank you.

Did this picture book help your child in some way?
If so, I would love to hear about it!

www.amazon.com/gp/product-review/B0D15X44LP

For other book titles, please visit:

www.fzwbooks.com

Connect with the Author

email: books@fzwbooks.com
facebook/instagram: @FZWbooks

About the Author

Dr. Fei Zheng-Ward is a clinical anesthesiologist who understands the apprehension patients (both adults and children) may have surrounding their upcoming surgery. Her goal in her medical books is to bring useful information to patients so they have a better understanding and appreciation of what happens leading up to, during, and after surgery. She wants readers to be more empowered to make informed decisions and to feel more at ease with their surgery.

As a practicing physician, she takes pride in being respected for her attention to detail, commitment to providing compassionate and personalized patient care, and strong presence in patient advocacy in the perioperative period for each of her patients. She understands the importance of physical and emotional well-being and advocates for patient autonomy.

In addition to her clinical practice, Dr. Zheng-Ward is actively involved in medical education and contributes to medical journals and state and national conferences.

She is an award-winning author for her book titled ***What to Expect and How to Prepare for Your Surgery***.

More about Dr. Fei Zheng-Ward:

* Board Certified Anesthesiologist

* Anesthesiology Residency Training at The Johns Hopkins Hospital in Baltimore, MD

* Master in Public Health (MPH) degree from Dartmouth Medical School in Hanover, NH

Books by the author

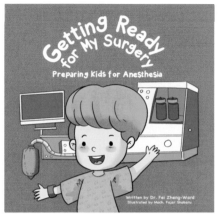

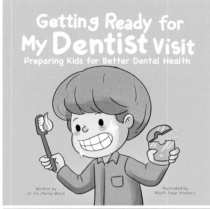

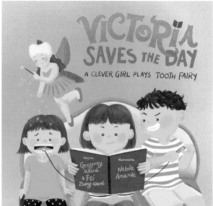

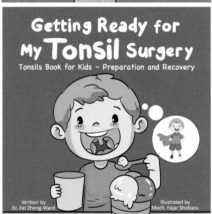

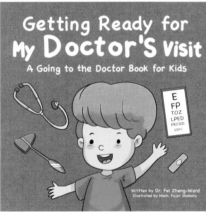

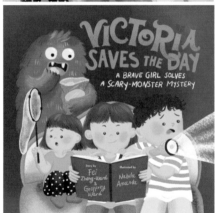

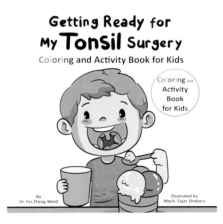

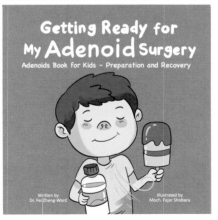

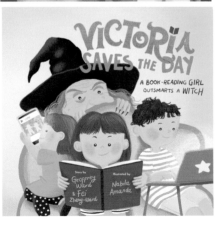

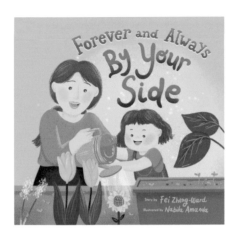

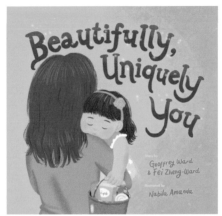

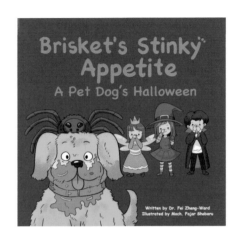

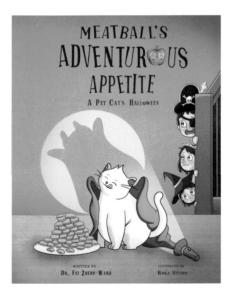

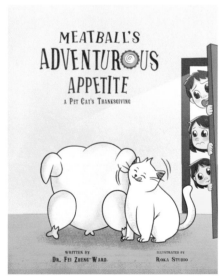

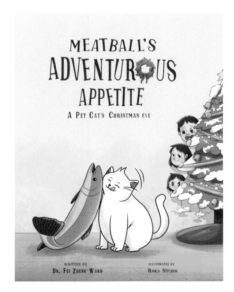

Follow the author for more upcoming titles.

Made in United States
Troutdale, OR
12/03/2024

25462302R00029